The Five Elements Healing Arts

Sub title: Food is the best medicine

By Jinho Lee

____

- Preface –

My memories of my childhood are filled with frequent migraines, stomach aches, allergies, back pain, etc. The illnesses and symptoms had no identifiable cause and generally ruined this period in my life. As I got older, I came to realize I was not alone in my struggles with random illnesses. Lots of people are affected by diseases for which there is no cure. As science and technology improve, many new things are discovered, but many remain a mystery. This is the limitation of technology. If you approach the human body armed with only scientific knowledge, your information will be incomplete and your results may not be ideal. Even medical doctors recognize the benefits of alternative treatments in healing patients. This is why some alternative methods are being adopted in hospitals.

Since I required frequent treatment as a child, I grew up interested in health and studied related topics such as acupressure, Shiatsu, Tui na, Sasang constitutional medicine, Ayurveda, Qi gong and meditation. Looking back, some were good and some were not. However, I can say that all of them helped me improve my knowledge. Over time, I dropped some and focused on the useful ones.

I returned to Korea in 2015 after several years in Australia and the United States. My constitution had improved over the years, but I still had random aches and pains. An acquaintance introduced me to a Korean traditional healer, who told me about the Five Elements healing method. I found the concepts to be quite logical and began to apply them to my body. The method was the best I had attempted by far and I was amazed by the results.

The Five Elements healing method was introduced by Chunsik Kim, who passed away in 1998. To provide a brief summary about him, he applied the entire method to his body and in the process, improved and modified the theory over his lifetime. Therefore, the final method is a testament to his spirit and his sacrifice. I salute him from the bottom of my heart.

One of the best parts about the Five Elements method is that it is simple and easy to understand. In addition, it works faster than other traditional methods if you follow the instructions properly. This guide draws from Chunsik Kim's teachings, his life and his book *O-hang Saengsik Yobeop* (Five elements raw food method, 1998), distilled through my experiences as a lifelong student of the martial and energy arts. I summarize the theory here in a format that is easy to digest with the hope that this method can help many people who are struggling with illness.

This method is powerful and practical. It will work for most internal issues, but is not aimed at treating injuries or wounds. Exercise good judgment when putting this method into practice.

Table of contents

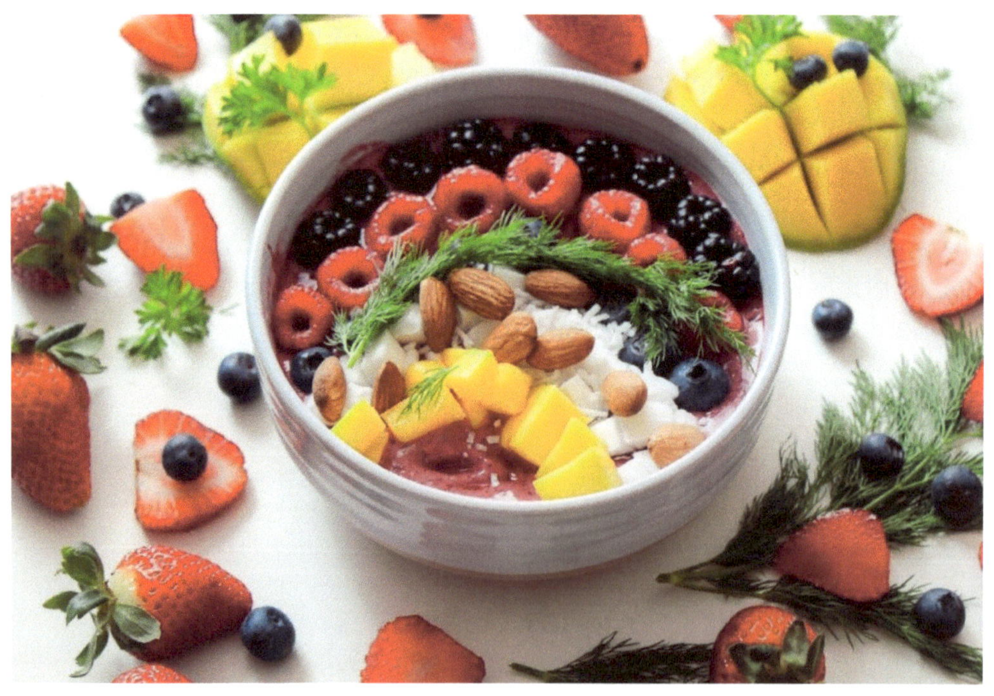

Chapter 1. The Theory of the Five Elements

The Five Elements Theory is based on ancient Chinese philosophy. Ancient Chinese physicians and scholars believed that everything in the world is composed of five elements which influence everything including tangibles like trees and buildings as well as intangibles like human personality and health. The elements are Fire, Earth, Metal, Water and Wood. These elements interact with each other in a continuous cycle of mutual creation and destruction.

A sixth aspect, *Sanghwa*, ties the five elements together. Though *Sanghwa* is not a physical organ, ancient Asians believed it was essential for humans. To break down the term, *Sang* means "each other" and *Hwa* means "fire". The term is best translated as "life force" and this aspect is made up of the Mind (*Simpo*) and the Spirit (*Samcho*, soul). We will explore the concept in more detail in Chapter 3.

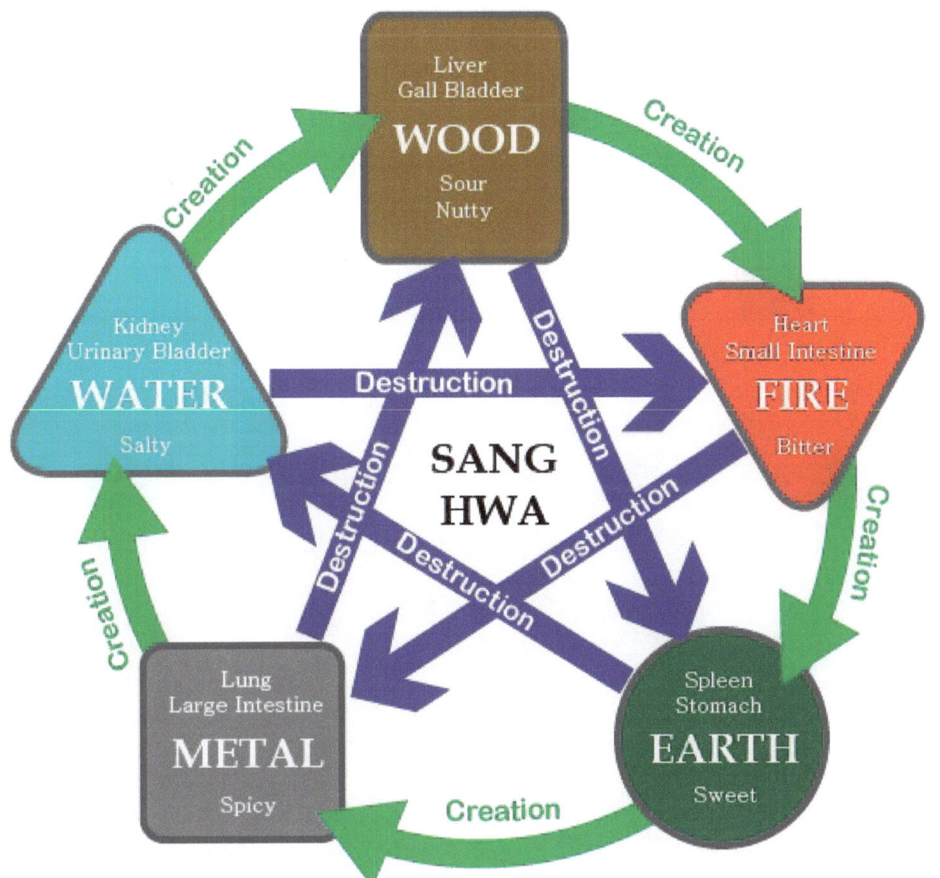

Each element is embodied by different organs in the human body as well as different tastes. You can heal yourself with food if you find the rule that applies to you in the above picture. For example, if you suddenly develop heart problems, it means you recently had too much or not enough bitter foods such as coffee, alcohol or turkey. Or you may have had too many salty foods such as chestnut, pork or tofu. In this situation, reducing salty foods and eating sour or nutty foods will help your heart recover. You may also need to increase or reduce your intake of bitter foods depending on your condition. The key is BALANCE and HARMONY.

Everyone is born with at least one strong element. Some people have strong hearts, which means they were born with fire as their strong element, making them fire types. The element a person is born with is the most important element to balance and harmonize and the strength of an individual in each element can change depending on diet.

Some people are mixed types. People strong in two elements such as Wood + Fire, Fire + Earth, Earth + Metal, Metal + Water, and Water + Wood are as common as those strong in a single element. Strength in three elements is possible as well, specifically, Wood + Fire + Earth, Fire + Earth + Metal, Earth + Metal + Water, Metal + Water + Wood, and Water + Wood + Fire. These kinds of people are not as common as the other two.

In order to heal yourself using the Five Elements, you first need to understand the underlying mechanism.

Chapter 2. Constitution Classification

This chapter will tell you about the organs and tastes for each element.

1) Wood

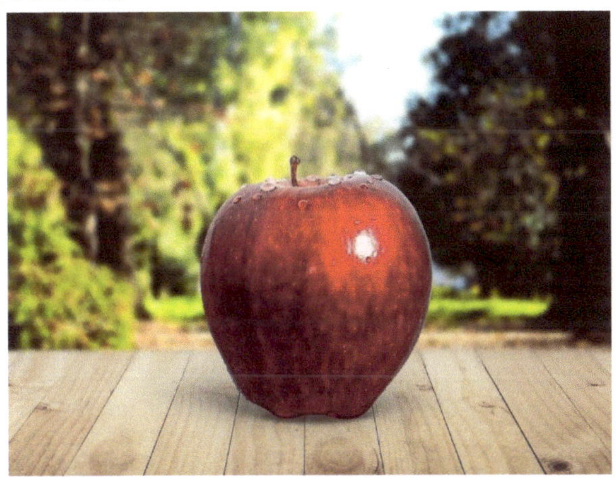

Organs: Liver, gall bladder.
Tastes: Sour and nutty.

Affected body parts and symptoms:
Liver, gall bladder, muscles, throat, tonsils, thyroid glands, hip joints, eyes, nails, feet, tears, migraines.

Foods for the wood type:
- Fruits: Strawberry, plum, grapes, apple, tangerine, pine nuts, walnut, peanut, sesame, perilla seeds, Japanese apricot, pineapple, cherry, Chinese quince, citron, pomegranate.
- Vegetables: Scallion, sour kimchi, sesame leaf.
- Meat products: Chicken, egg, quail, animal liver, gall bladder.
- Seasonings: Vinegar, sesame oil, citric acid, raisins, perilla oil.
- Beverages: Orange juice, citron tea, peanut tea, cider, schisandra tea.

2) Fire

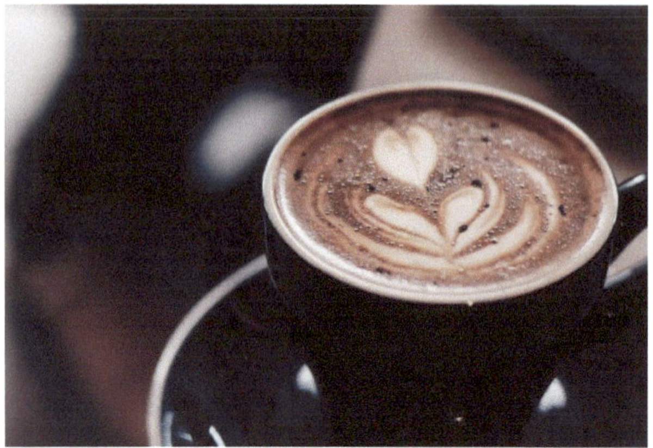

Organs: Heart, small intestine.
Tastes: Bitter.

Affected body parts and symptoms:
Heart, small intestine, blood, blood vessels, elbows, arms, shoulder blades, face, tongue, sweat, pimples, sciatica.

Foods for the fire type:
- Fruits: Apricot, grapefruit, ginkgo, sunflower seeds.
- Vegetables: Unripe hot pepper, lettuce, crown daisy, bellflower, bonnet bellflower, chard, celery, ganoderma lucidum (reishi mushroom), Korean lettuce, shepherd's purse, wild edible greens, dandelion, motherwort, mugwort, seasoned aster.
- Meat products: Goat, deer, animal heart, chitterlings, sparrow, grasshopper, turkey.
- Seasonings: Alcohol, black bean paste, chocolate, cottonseed oil.
- Beverages: Black tea, green tea, coffee, ganoderma lucidum (reishi mushroom) tea, mugwort tea.

3) Earth

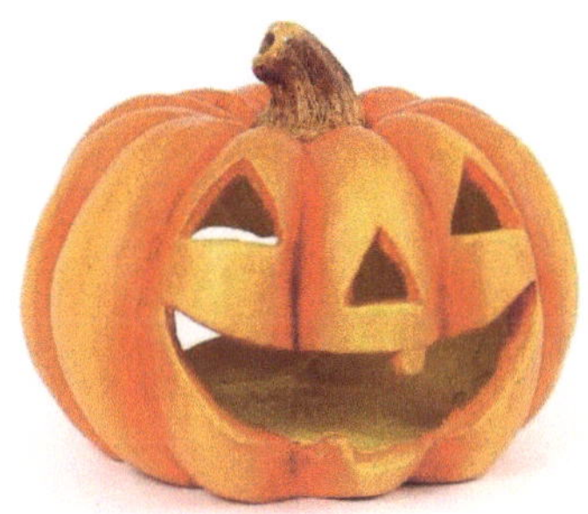

Organs: Spleen, stomach.
Tastes: Sweet.

Affected body parts and symptoms:
Spleen, stomach, pancreatitis, duodenum, mouth, lip, breast,
thighs, knee joint, heel, nose, fat, skin oiliness, overweight.

Foods for the earth type:
- Fruits: Oriental melon, persimmon, jujube, arrowroot, sweet
potato, pumpkin.
- Vegetables: Parsley, ginseng, licorice, lotus root, spinach, sweet
potato stem.
- Meat products: Beef, rabbit, crucian carp, chitterlings, pancreas.
- Seasonings: Sugar, honey, toffee, toffee oil, jam, butter, glucose,
margarine.
- Beverages: Ginseng tea, arrowroot tea, jujube tea, goji berry tea,
eucommia ulmoides (du zhong) tea, sweet rice drink.

4) Metal

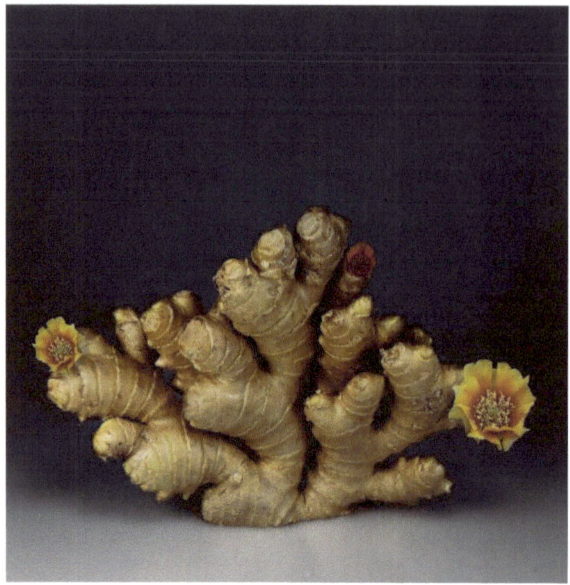

Organs: Lungs, large intestine.
Tastes: Spicy.

Affected body parts and symptoms:

Lungs, large intestine, skin, nose, body hair, chest, wrist, forearm, anus, diarrhea, allergies, snot, conception vessel.

Foods for the metal type:
- Fruits: Peach, pear, cinnamon.
- Vegetables: Green onion, garlic, pepper, Korean pickled-peel garlic, radish, cabbage, onion, squill.
- Meat products: Fish, shells, animal lungs, horse.
- Seasonings: Red pepper powder or paste, mustard, black pepper, peppermint, wasabi, ginger, garlic flower stalk.
- Beverages: Job's tears tea, milk, ginger tea, cinnamon fruit punch, cinnamon tea.

5) Water

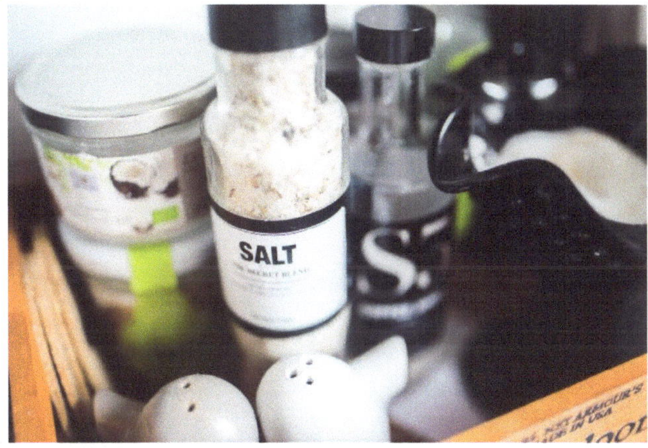

Organs: Kidney, urinary bladder.
Tastes: Salty.

Affected body parts and symptoms:

Kidneys, urinary bladder, adrenal gland, genitals, womb, ear, teeth, waist, buttocks, ankles, bone, marrow, tendon, calf, hair, saliva, nerves, osteoporosis.

Foods for the metal type:
- Fruits: Watermelon, chestnut.
- Vegetables: Seaweed, laver, green laver, tangleweed, flax, various ascidiacea (sea squirts).
- Meat products: Pork, sea slug, thick beef soup, anchovy, animal kidneys, frog, snake, earthworm.
- Seasonings: Salt, bamboo salt, soy sauce, miso, tofu, salted seafood, cheese.
- Beverages: Soy milk, matcha tea.

6) *Sanghwa*

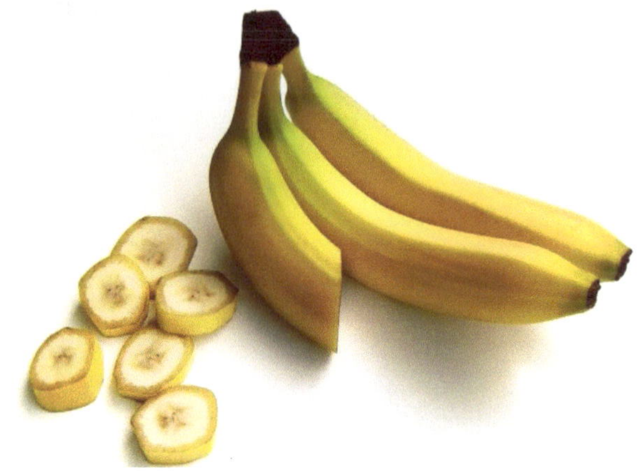

Organs: *Simpo* (mind), *samcho* (spirit).
Tastes: Astringent.

Affected body parts and symptoms:

Mind, spirit, emotions, disease resistance, respiratory tract, gullet, prostate, metabolism, nervousness, stress, hand, shoulder joints, thyroid gland, depression, insomnia.

Foods for the *sanghwa* type:
- Fruits: Tomato, banana, potato, taro, almond, acorn.
- Vegetables: Bean sprouts, mushroom, cucumber, carrot, cabbage, bracken, edible shoots of a fatsia (Japanese aralia), eggplant, burdock, agar, mallow (a type of hibiscus), bamboo shoots, pine mushroom, green bean sprouts.
- Meats: Mutton, duck, pupa, squid, pollack fish (note this fish is different from pollock), duck eggs, pheasant.
- Seasonings: Tomato ketchup, mayonnaise, royal jelly.
- Beverages: Yogurt, cola, cocoa, bine/hop tea, aloe, ion drinks.

Chapter 3. Sanghwa (Simpo and Samcho)

Sanghwa is an unknown concept in the West (it is barely known in modern Asian society as well). This chapter is dedicated to explaining *Sanghwa, Simpo* (mind) and *Samcho* (spirit).

Sanghwa represents the life force of an individual. At the right amount, it helps ensure proper circulation of *chi* (energy) and blood in the body. However, too much *Sanghwa* can cause a person to age too quickly and can lead to illness and death. This is why the ancient Chinese healers used *chi* to control *Sanghwa*.

Simpo and *Samcho* are responsible for regulating the balance of vitality and the immune system in humans and are based around the concept of yin and yang. *Simpo* and *Samcho* are related to stress and the mind and can easily block the *chi* and blood circulation when not in harmony. They are not visible, but they are very important parts of our health and control our overall wellbeing, immunity, and direct connections to the mind.

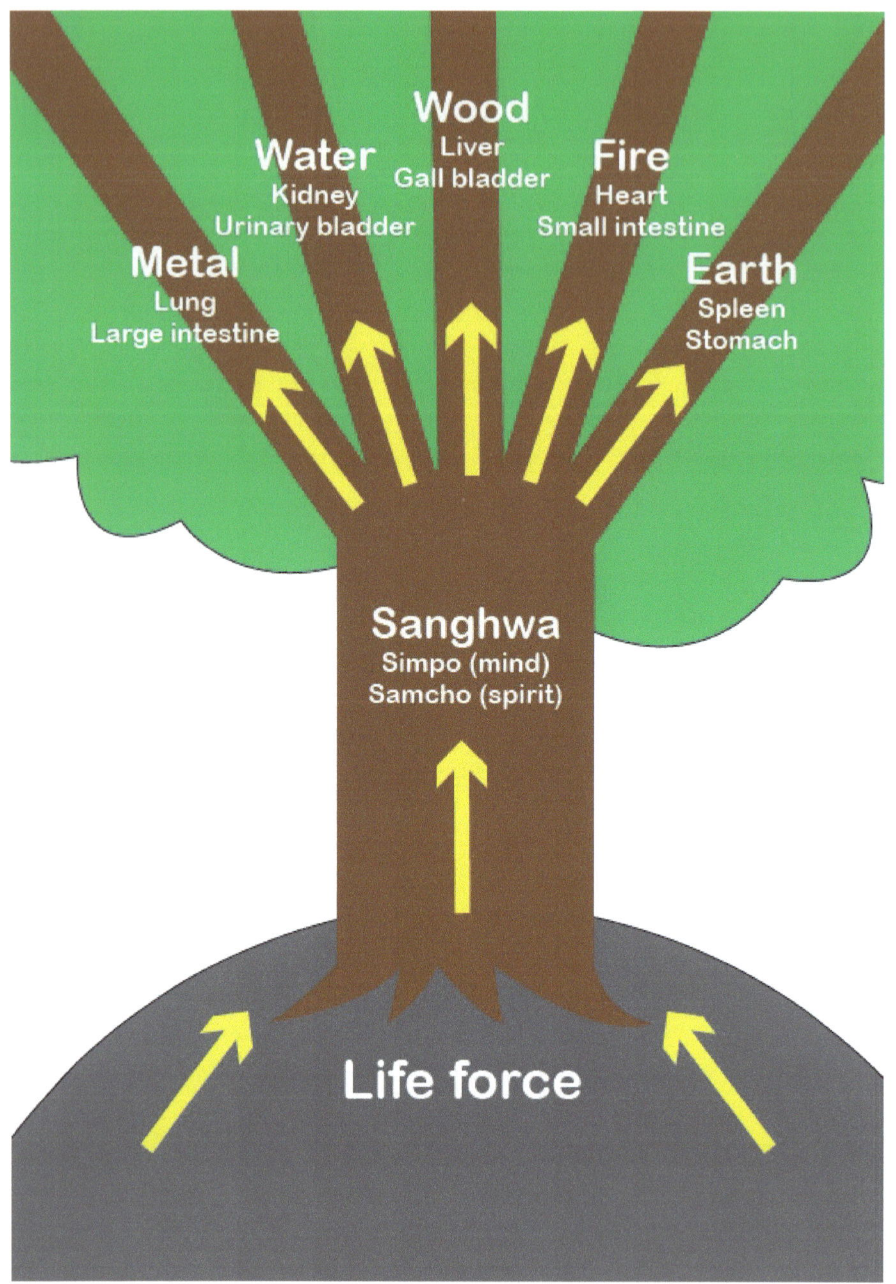

Let's assume the trunk of the tree is *Simpo* and *Samcho*. If the energy of *Simpo* and *Samcho* is blocked, less energy is supplied to the organs and eventually the body becomes ill. Therefore, *Simpo* and *Samcho* are the center and starting point of the body through which the life force and energy passes.

There is actually a point where the meridian of *Simpo* and *Samcho* converge. If you drill through this section, you can use the energy, which is normally difficult to access. Continuing with the tree analogy, trees absorb nutrition from their roots and transfer the nutrients to their branches and leaves. However, when the path is blocked, the branches are less nourished. The energy of the body, the vitality, the path through which this energy travels; this is all *Simpo* and *Samcho*. They provide energy to the organs.

If blood circulation to *Simpo* and *Samcho* is blocked, you can only use about 50% of your energy. This blockage will affect the other major parts of the body, causing the whole body to deteriorate. It is important to take good care of your energy to prevent *Simpo* and *Samcho* blockage in the body due to mental problems such as nervousness and stress.

Chapter 4. Personality Classification

Each element has its own characteristics and everybody has a different personality. This chapter will tell you about the changes in personality according to the status of each element.

1) Wood

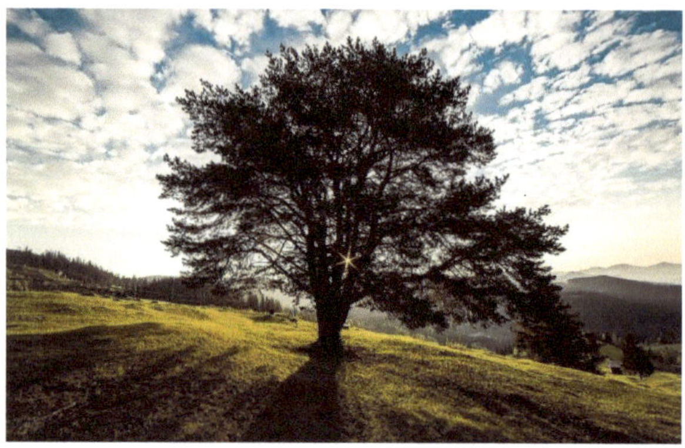

- Benign
- Good at color discrimination
- Resourceful
- Poetic
- Literary
- Educational
- Warm hearted
- Mild
- Administrative
- Writer
- Not strict
- Sensitive
- Positive about everything
- Pursues growth
- Good explainer
- Honest
- Generous

The personality in a weak condition:

- Paranoid
- Yelling
- Quick to anger
- Violent
- Craves sour and nutty taste
- Sighs often
- Health is worse in spring and at dawn
- Makes decisions carelessly
- Dislikes wind
- Teases others
- Mean
- Uses offensive words
- Smells of sour and burning hair
- Sarcastic
- Ignores people
- Has poor judgment
- Not submissive
- Hurts others

Physical subjective symptoms:

- Pain in meridian
- Pain in liver
- Muscle pain
- Muscle spasms
- Gets cramps easily
- Coating on the tongue
- Goose bumps
- Shrinking of the genitals
- Back pain
- Joint pain
- Hepatitis A and C
- Symptoms on nails
- Liver cancer
- Migraines, Stiff throat
- Gallstones
- Pleurisy
- Convulsion
- Squinting

- Phlegm
- Neck gets thicker
- Sleep talking
- Teeth grinding
- Sleepwalking
- Stomach ache in the morning
- Tears
- Bed-wetting
- Stiff skin

2) Fire

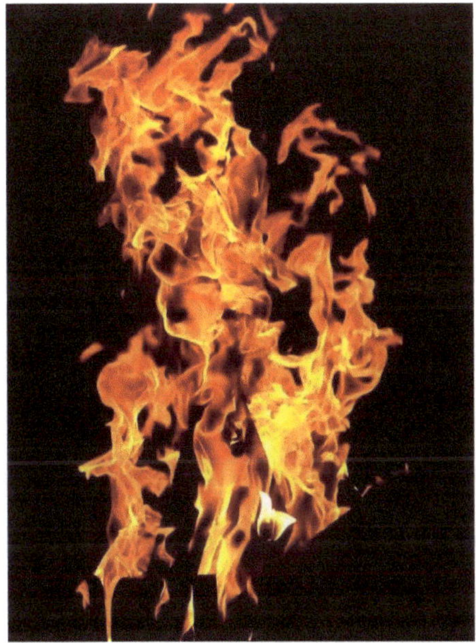

The personality in a healthy condition:
- Well-mannered
- Places great importance on order
- Cheerful
- Vivacious
- Inquisitive
- Brave
- Keen sixth sense
- Artistic
- Loves sports
- Sensual
- Considerate
- Emotionally expressive
- Generous
- Easygoing
- Fearless
- Risk taker

The personality in a weak condition:
- Laughs too much
- Gets angry easily
- Easily surprised

- Rude
- Gets ill in the morning and in the summer
- Craves bitter and burning taste
- Aggressive
- Desperate
- Explosive
- Avoids heat
- Bitter and burning smell
- Pounding heart
- Mournful
- Extravagant
- Gaudy
- Arrogant
- Short tempered
- Distractive
- One-sided love

Physical subjective symptoms:
- Bloodshot eyes
- Pounding heart
- Red cheeks
- Heavy sweating
- Often thirsty
- Joint pain
- Shoulder blade pain
- Sciatica
- Stammers
- Face edema
- High blood pressure
- Valvular disease
- Arteriosclerosis
- Myocardial infarction
- Solar plexus pain
- Small lung capacity
- Hiccup often
- Internal bleeding
- Vascular abnormalities
- Hip pain
- Recurrent miscarriage

- Sterility
- Menstrual pain

3) Earth

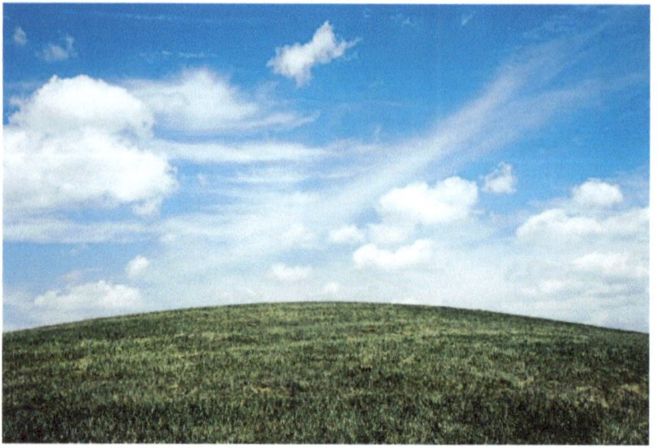

The personality in a healthy condition:
- Accurate
- Thorough
- Certain
- Single-minded
- Submissive
- Reliable
- Focused
- Harmonized
- Solid
- Self-interested
- Gentle
- Hates complicated things

The personality in a weak condition:
- Delusional
- Gets ill in the afternoon and in late summer
- Deep thinking
- Lying
- Doubtful
- Morbid jealousy
- Dull
- Lazy
- Repetitive talk and action
- Burdensome
- Burps often
- Craves sweets

- Festered smell
- Hates humidity
- Complains a lot

Physical subjective symptoms:
- Issues on mouth and lips
- Facial nerve paralysis
- Loose mouth
- Twisted mouth
- Forehead pain
- Lower teeth pain
- Easily bruised
- Knee joint pain
- Gastric ulcer
- Sour stomach
- Breast issues
- Obesity
- Crack in the heel
- Easily tired
- Gastric cancer
- Spleen cancer
- Trembling
- Gloomy
- Stiff tongue
- Bad breath
- Oily skin
- Diabetic
- Red nose
- Bulimia nervosa
- Lack of leukocyte

4) Metal

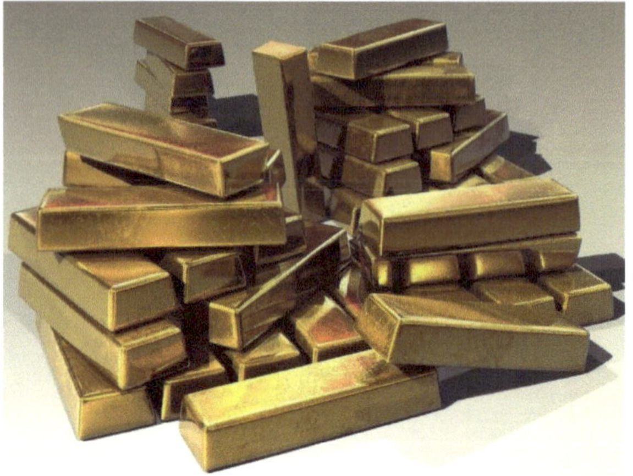

The personality in a healthy condition:
- Strong leadership
- Good control abilities
- Loyal
- Law-abiding
- Loves routine
- Uniformity
- Competitive
- Ambitious
- Successful
- Good at organizing
- Proud
- Interested in moral self-development
- Respectful
- Unbiased
- Honest
- Rational
- Leader
- Loyal

The personality in a weak condition:
- Pessimistic
- Sad
- Depressed
- Demotivated
- Suicidal

- Too compassionate
- Sneezes easily
- Gets ill in the evening and in autumn
- Craves spicy and fishy foods
- Fishy smell on the body
- Hates dryness
- Tearful voice
- Dictator
- Whining
- Conceited
- Unreliable
- Controlling
- Extreme
- Feels pity for strangers

Physical subjective symptoms:
- Rhinitis
- Nose allergies
- Nosebleed
- Snot
- Nasal congestion
- Lung disease
- Pulmonary tuberculosis
- Lung cancer
- Colon cancer
- Rectal cancer
- Wrist joint pain
- Wrist arthritis
- Sneezing
- Small lung capacity
- Cough
- Asthma
- Cecum issues
- Cataract
- Feeling of fullness in the chest
- Constipation
- Hemorrhoids
- Anal fistula
- Colitis

- Food poisoning
- Alopecia or hairiness
- Frequent diarrhea
- Skin diseases
- Skin cancer
- Allergies

5) Water

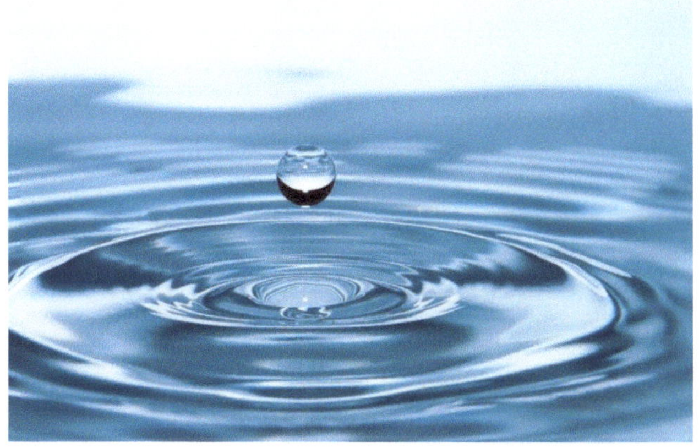

The personality in a healthy condition:
- Strong stamina
- Patient
- Wise
- Good at math
- Good at science
- Mechanical
- Strong virility
- Introverted
- Development oriented
- Suggests new ideas
- Studious
- Expansive
- Modest
- Good at keeping secrets
- Constructive opinions
- Creates a positive atmosphere
- Lots of ideas
- Reticent
- Persistent

The personality in a weak condition:
- Negative
- Contradictive
- Revolutionary
- Exaggerates pain

- Complains about sad plight
- Only eats and plays
- Makes excuses
- Unreliable
- Fearful
- Gets ill at night and in the winter
- Craves salty food
- Too shy
- Passive
- Stubborn

Physical subjective symptoms:
- Split hairs
- Hair loss
- Tinnitus (ringing in the ears)
- Deafness
- Tympanitis (inflamed ear drum)
- Gloomy
- Loose chin
- Edema
- Kidney hypertension
- Yawns often
- Lack of appetite
- Sterile
- Larynx pain
- Pain in the crook of the knee
- Calf pain
- Lower back pain
- Speaking in a groan
- Eyes seem to pop out
- Bone infection
- Smells rotten
- Kidney stones
- Protein in urine
- Kidney cancer
- Bladder cancer
- Drools
- Anemic
- Near-sightedness

- Far-sightedness

6) *Sanghwa*

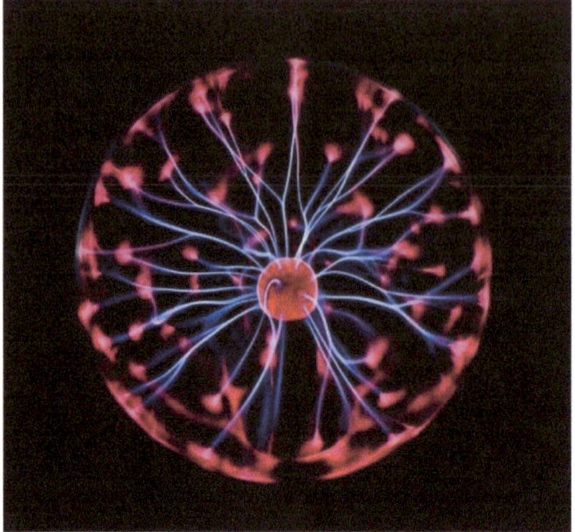

The personality in a healthy condition:
- Versatile
- Masterful
- Acts according to the circumstances
- Intelligent
- Everybody's friend
- Calm
- Strong life force
- Strong immune system
- Agile
- Energetic
- Good immune system
- Hardy
- Mediator
- Empathetic
- Long lived
- Neither lazy nor hasty
- Harmonized, gentle
- Flexible
- Adapts well to new environments

The personality in a weak condition:
- Uneasy
- Anxious
- Nervous

- Depression
- Short tempered
- Shy
- Easily offended and irritated
- Embarrassed
- Trickster
- Show off
- Brown noser
- Mischief-maker
- Unfocused
- Bustling
- Reduced immunity
- Tired
- Enervated
- Sobs
- Gets ill during the change of season
- Hates sunshine

Physical subjective symptoms:
- Numb hand and foot
- Arthritis of the hands
- Eczema
- Insomnia
- Sweat and heat on the palm
- Dry, cracked palms
- Shoulder joint pain
- Shoulder arthritis
- Heavy shoulders
- Chest pain
- Dry mouth
- Swollen throat and tonsils
- Lymphatic fluid issues, lymph cancer
- Arrhythmia
- Coccyx pain
- Menstrual issues
- Bladder issues
- Nervous indigestion
- Recurrent miscarriage
- Low blood platelet count

- Swollen prostate

Chapter 5. The shape of each type of element and the appropriate treatment

Each type of element has a specific shape and a person's strong element or elements is reflected in their body. This may be in the shape of the head or the shape of the entire body. To confirm the shape of the head, it is necessary to check the forehead as well, because hair usually covers the face and can make it difficult to see the actual shape.

The size of each organ varies depending on the element type and all types have different features. This chapter will tell you about all of the above.

1) Wood

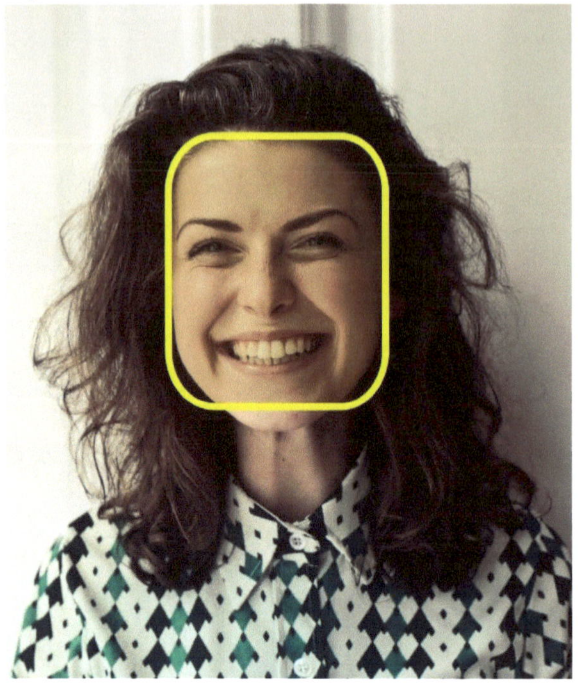

The shape of the wood type is rectangular.

The size of the organs:
- Liver, gall bladder: Big
- Spleen, stomach: Small
- Lung, large intestine: Small

Treatments:
- Neck exercise
- Flank exercise
- Foot exercise
- Hip turn
- Eye exercise

Features:
- Thin
- Long
- Slippery
- Tense

2) **Fire**

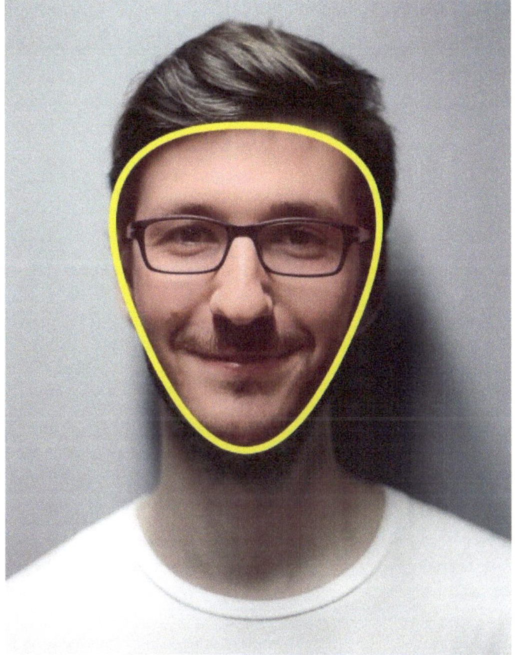

The shape of the fire type is an inverted triangle.

The size of the organs:
- Heart, small intestine: Big
- Lung, large intestine: Small
- Kidney, urinary bladder: Small

Treatments:
- Shoulder exercise
- Push-ups
- Facial massage
- Tongue exercise

Features:
- Soft
- Bony
- Bursting with emotions

3) Earth

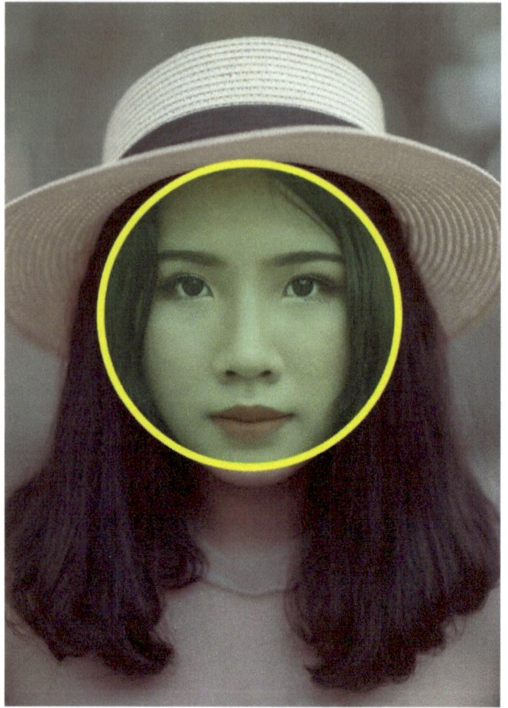

The shape of the earth type is circular.

The size of the organs:
- Spleen, stomach: Big
- Kidney, urinary bladder: Small
- Liver, gall bladder: Small

Treatments:
- Knee exercise
- Sit-ups

Features:
- Thick
- Wide
- Short
- Slow

4) Metal

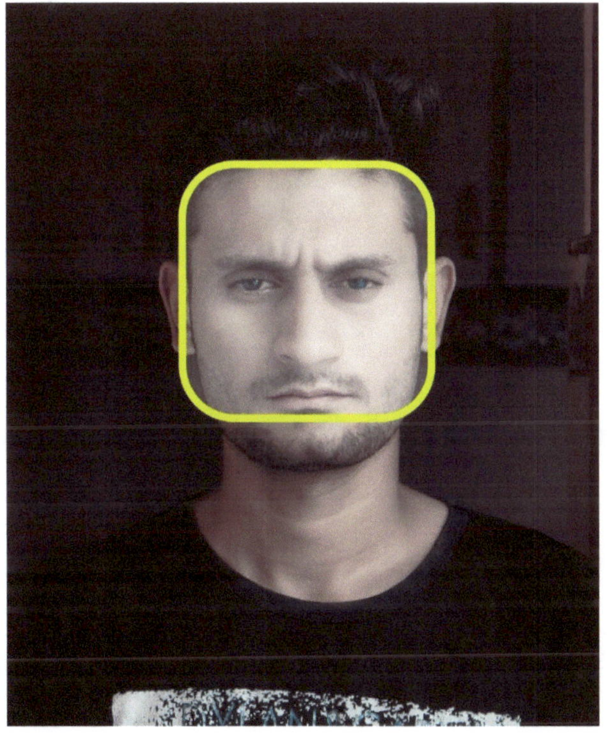

The shape of the metal type is square.

The size of the organs:
- Lungs, large intestine: Big
- Liver, gall bladder: Small
- Heart, small intestine: Small

Treatments:
- Wrist exercises
- Slow breathing

Features:
- Thick
- Wide
- Short
- Stoic

5) Water

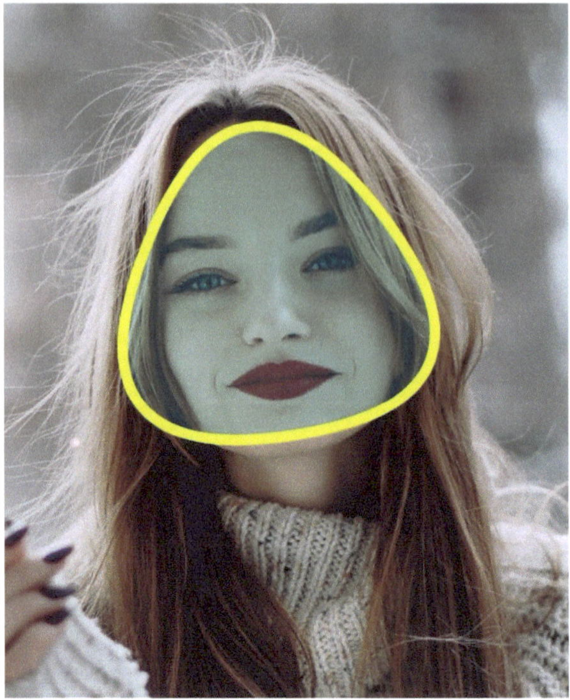

The shape of the water type is triangular.

The size of the organs:
- Kidneys, urinary bladder: Big
- Heart, small intestine: Small
- Spleen, stomach: Small

Treatments:
- Ankle exercises
- Waist turn
- Standing on the toes

Features:
- Slippery
- Solid
- Thick and rich
- Staunch

6) *Sanghwa*

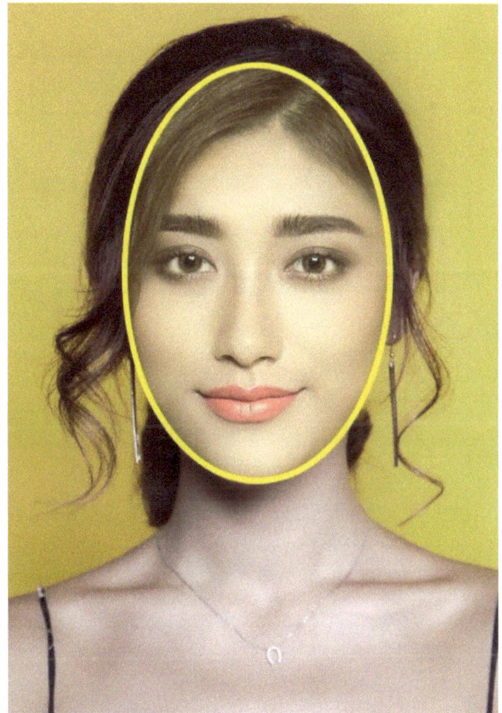

The shape of the *Sanghwa* type is oval.

The size of the organs:
- *Simpo* (mind), *Samcho* (spirit): Big
- Other organs: Balanced

Treatments:
- Quality time with trusted confidants
- Finger exercises
- Clapping
- Repeatedly opening and closing the hands

Features:
- Thin
- Long
- Soft
- Bony

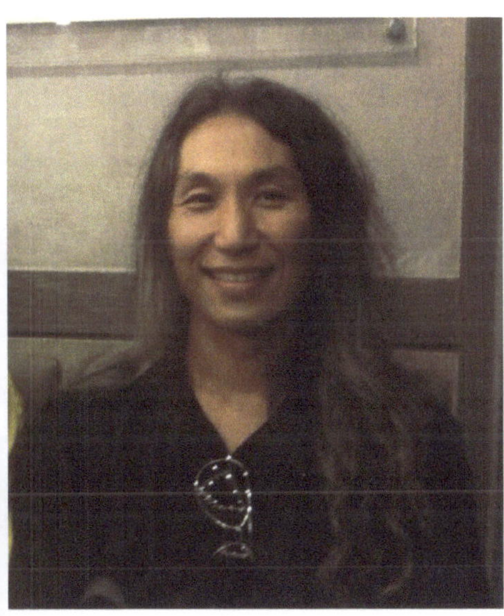

About the author

Jinho Lee was born in South Korea. He was born weak and struggled with many illnesses. He began practicing external martial arts when he was thirteen and switched to internal arts at twenty nine. He also studied I Ching, acupuncture, acupressure, Shiatsu, Tui na, and natural therapies. Jinho moved to Australia in 2008 and to the USA in 2012. During this period, he realized that the skills he had learned were valuable. His purpose is to share what he has learned in the hopes that it will help others improve their health.

Other books by the author

2015, The Key to the Internal Arts

<u>**Biography**</u>

- 1984, Studied Tanglang Quan under Master Deok-Kang Lee

- 1990, Studied Hapkido under Master Dongnam Park

- 1993, Studied Taekwondo in military life

- 1994, Hapkido Instructor

- 1999, Studied Karate and Aikido at a martial arts community

- 2002, Studied Kendo, Security guard martial arts, Shaolin Quan, Qi Gong, and Tai Chi Quan under Master Chang-Kuk Oh

- 2003, Studied Baji Quan, Baguazhang and Qi Gong under Master Namseong Kim

- 2004, Studied Yang and Chen style Tai Chi Quan, Yinyang Baguazhang, Nei Gong, Dayan (Wild Goose) Qi Gong, and Xinyi Liuhe Quan under Master Min-Young Jung

- 2007, Internal Kung Fu, Tai Chi and Qi Gong head instructor, Seoul, Korea

- 2008, Internal Kung Fu, Self-defense, Tai Chi and Qi Gong head instructor, Melbourne, Australia

- 2009, Tai Chi instructor, Melbourne, Australia

- 2010, Tai Chi instructor, Melbourne, Australia

- 2018, Studied Chen Style Tai Chi Quan under Master Wonil Jeong